BUSY COUPLES SEX COUPONS

EASY COUPONS TO MAKE THE TIME

J.L. Silver

TEAR COUPONS OUT TO REDEEM

This coupon is for one blowjob, while I sit in my office chair doing work.

Back Side Of Coupon

This coupon is for one Oral Pleasure session for her, while she gets some work done.

Back Side Of Coupon

This coupon is for one quickie before work in the morning, 20 minutes is all you get.

Back Side Of Coupon

This coupon is for one night that we both have off to go to a hotel room or in our dining room of drinks, dinner, candles, dancing, and rough wild sex that last 2 hours.

Back
Side
Of
Coupon

This coupon is for one session of the 69 position in the middle of the night.

Back
Side
Of
Coupon

This coupon is for one blowjob, while he is eating dinner. Multi-Task at its best.

Back
Side
Of
Coupon

This coupon is for one bowl of cerel, while he gives her oral pleasure in bed

Back Side Of Coupon

Fast, Quick, Rough Dirty Sex. I need it now and I need it fast. You better be quick.

Back Side Of Coupon

This coupon is for sex in the shower. Soap each other up and have a little fun.

Back Side Of Coupon

This coupon is for doggystyle sex, but you both get to eat a sandwhich during it.

Kitchen tables work wonders.

Back
Side
Of
Coupon

Buy some virbrating thongs for her and at your next buisness function together give him the remote. You will want to rip his cloths off by the time it is over.

Back Side Of Coupon

This coupon is for one whole day of relaxation and sex. Eat, nap, sex, eat nap sex, watch tv, sex, read, sex, games, sex. You get the idea. This is a sex day. Make it worth it you have earned it.

Back
Side
Of
Coupon

I love you Forever And Always

To:

From: